Paths –

A Primer for

Ladies-of-a-Certain-Age

A Workbook for the Road Ahead

By

Elizabeth J. Wheeler

LCA Press Grand Junction, Colorado

www.ladiesofacertainage.com

Cover Designer: Joyce Cerritti

ISBN: 9798713829490
Imprint: Independently published

CONTENTS

FORWARD

What a jolt I had as a woman approaching retirement age. It would have been a shock to my system even if I had never worked outside the home. Even though I had planned for retirement, I needed to prepare better. I decided to share with you much of what I learned. This book will help you navigate the road ahead.

When I was nearing retirement, there was no "primer," if you will, for this time of life that I could get my hands on, and there was no way my parents or American society, for that matter, could have equipped me. Life had changed dramatically from the time I was born, shortly after the end of World War II, to the present time. My parents, Robert and Rose Wheeler, had given me a good upbringing. They impressed upon me their ethics of valuing family, education, and religion. We had a lovely home in one of Denver's new developments. My folks insisted I take shorthand and typing in high school "in case something happened to my future husband." Thank goodness they gave me an opportunity to go on to college, "a great place for finding a man to take care of her," was their thinking. (I did find that man and somehow ended up with a degree in the chaos of the 1960s. I didn't know any divorced people back then and would have been aghast if I looked in the future and saw my marriage dissolve after over a quarter of a century.) Then, I dreamed that, when I got to this age, I would be happily married for many years, have many grandchildren, live in an old bungalow close to my favorite park, and prepare Sunday dinners for family and friends.

I know my dream, or a variation of it, is shared by many American women. However, where we thought we would be at this stage of life and where we are is shocking in their differences.

Sure, I had planned for retirement financially, and I knew I wanted to play lots of golf, have a home on the Western Slope of Colorado, and travel. But, I didn't have a clue what was ahead of transitioning from a female executive to a retiree. I had no idea I would become invisible and not be valued much by American society.

In many ways, this book is a result of a blog titled "Ladies-of-a-Certain-Age," which I started writing shortly after retiring. The blog's purpose is to provide resources, information, support, and advocacy for one of the largest, wealthiest, and most powerful groups in America, females born between 1946 to 1964 in the Baby Boom generation. It is an outgrowth of my experience. I state in the About section of the website ladiesofacertainage.com: There comes a time in an American woman's life—somewhere around the age of 50—where she becomes invisible:

- Businesses no longer market to her.
- The fashion industry forsakes her.
- Television does not portray her, and radio does not broadcast her.

- Social and print media do not know her.

- Men and her children have forgotten her.

- Politicians certainly don't mention her.

- Yet she represents one of America's wealthiest, most powerful, and largest groups.

After writing almost 100 Ladies-of-a-Certain-Age blog posts, it occurred to me that it might be helpful if I wrote a simple workbook for women who were starting to recognize themselves as older, a primer—as school books used to be called—when we were in grade school about this time of life. So this book is for women about to retire, women who have lost their way in retirement or never knew which way to go, older women in the divorce process or about to be divorced, and widows. Women can go through it individually or in groups. A book club, study program, or a class could use it. Because women have cooperatively worked together throughout the ages and gained insights and support from one another, I feel it is best to go through this workbook in a group setting. In the addendum, I have provided suggested guidelines for group discussions.

The six chapters address the most critical questions that come up over and over again at this time of life:

1) Who am I now?

2) What lies ahead?

3) How do I deal with health changes?

4) Where does money come into all of this?

5) Why and when may I need different housing?

6) Will I have a purpose?

Each chapter has vital information, helpful, practical hints, and—of all things!—suggested homework, which I intend to be fun and insightful. The resources at the end of the book provide further reading, including a list of some of my relevant blog posts.

ACKNOWLEDGEMENTS

Many Thanks

When I did retire, I took a class from Denver's Academy for Lifelong Learning entitled "New Challenges for Women Over 60," taught by Elinor Miller Greenberg, PhD., a member of Colorado's Women's Hall of Fame. During the six-week class, I learned much about what my life would become, enjoyed lively discussions with my 60 classmates, and found many of the course exercises fascinating. I've included two in the second chapter: an expectations chart for the latter third of life and the anchors-in-life circle. This class contributed to my curiosity about why older American women are ignored, sparked my indignation, and, in 2013, propelled me to start writing a blog for this age group and increase the image of these invisible, powerful, and dynamic women.

When I moved to Colorado's Western Slope, I became aware of how little instruction and resources there were for older women in this less-populated area of the state. With Dr. Greenberg's support, I designed a class similar to hers for the local community college. I am deeply indebted to the experts I brought in for specific class topics: Linda Eden-Wallace, CFP; Martha Newman, Senior Real Estate Specialist; and Yvonne Barron, wellness instructor.

While I enjoyed developing material for the class and writing this book, I decided not to be a college instructor. I wanted to do other things in my life. I recognize how important it is for women entering this stage of life to get information about the numerous changes they are likely to experience. I hope such a class will be developed in the future.

I want to thank Gail Phillips, Ann Repka, and Debbie Peterson for reviewing and critiquing the book shortly before it was published. I respect their thoughtful analysis and the life experiences they brought to this review.

If you like this book, please post a review on Amazon and let your friends know about it on social media. Because ratings and reviews —even just a word or two—draw new readers to a possibly valuable experience. If you feel at a loss, here are some one-sentence reviews, which you are welcome to use verbatim:

"I'm so happy I discovered this excellent book at an important time in my life."

"I thought I had planned for retirement, but this book goes beyond the health and financial information I had."

Thank you! More positive reviews and word-of-mouth mean I can spend more time writing.

Elizabeth J. Wheeler
Grand Junction, Colorado

Chapter One

WHO AM I NOW?

You've Come a Long Way, Baby!
Virginia Slims

You are a crone, dear, a post-menopausal woman with tons of life experience. I call us Boomer Babes. We come from that unique American generation born just after World War II and up to the Gulf of Tonkin Resolution, passed by the US Congress in 1964.

This chapter covers three topics:

1) Summary of who we are now.
2) Where we came from.
3) How we got to where we are today.

Summary of who we are now

Who are Boomer Babes? Here's a quick general overview:

–Children are grown.

–Many of us have grandchildren and great-grandkids.

–We're retired or nearing retirement.

–There are no more rungs to climb at the "job."

–Generally, because we have worked with groups all our lives, unlike men, we are naturally comparative, not competitive.

–Our "girlfriends" are important to us.

–We out-survive men.

–Over 30 percent of us are single now, and we make our own decisions.

–Many of us are college-educated and have held management or professional positions.

−We have money−from our earnings, shared marital assets,
inherited wealth from parents, in-laws, and husbands.

−Many of us are healthy with life expectancies in the 90s if cancer,
heart disease, or something else doesn't strike.

−We have time to pursue old passions and explore new ones.

But, before we can answer the question, who am I now, we need to look back at where we came from: our journey to this incredible time in our lives.

Where we came from

The experience for those women born between 1946-1954 and those between 1955-1964 varies. Life for the second group accelerated because of the ever-increasing change in American society due to technology, medical breakthroughs, and the feminist liberation movement.

For example, the first group of women often recalls with joy the day their family got a black-and-white television set. The second group needs help remembering black-and-white television shows and just having one television in the house. Likewise, the first group of women giggles when they remember the family telephone party line. The second group remembers either themselves or their lucky friends having a pink princess phone in their bedrooms.

Both groups grew up in a very different world than their mothers. Almost every aspect of their lives was unlike their mothers, who had no way to prepare their daughters for their adult years. Moreover, virtually every American institution changed from the 1920s through the 1930s when their mothers grew up.

I wish I could say that today's older American women are as revered as they were in ancient Irish or American Indian cultures. Both of those were matriarchal cultures. Women held power, political leadership, moral authority, social privilege, and control. I wish I could also say older American women today are as valued as women in many parts of the world for their knowledge, experiences, and just because they are older women.

In this country, life for women of all ages began to change in World War II. Many women started to work outside the home since they needed to fill jobs previously held by men who went off to war. When the war was over, many women returned to their homes because men came back to their previous employment. But, something began to change for women because the family structure started to alter. Grown children and their families began moving away from small towns and farms to metropolitan areas.

In the cities, more women worked outside of the home. They often were nurses, teachers, secretaries, or shop employees. Families were moving to new housing developments, necessitating a car. In their new automobiles, families took summer vacations and traveled outside of their state on newly built interstate highways. Unlike today, divorce was low.

Supposedly, women's domestic work was getting more manageable because of the new electric appliances such as washing machines, dryers, dishwashers, and vacuum cleaners—convenience foods–from cake mixes to TV dinners–began to appear on the grocery shelves.

Then, the sixties came! Gloria Steinem published *Ms. Magazine*, the feminist movement gained speed, and many more women started working outside their homes. Cigarette manufacturer Phillip Morris capitalized on society's change by introducing a new product geared toward women. The new Virginia Slims cigarette tagline, "You've Come A Long Way, Baby," epitomized what had happened to American women.

It was a time when the first group of today's ladies of a certain age were teenagers. Many of these girls went off to college, burned their bras, started taking those new birth-control pills, and demanded equality.

<u>How we got to where we are today</u>

As ladies of a certain age, we do not have role models from the women who brought us into this world. Our generation, the Baby Boomers, live longer than our mothers, generally have secured more education than they did, and have worked for a good part of our lives. Thanks to the Women's Movement and birth-control pills, our lives have been very different from our dear ol' moms.

So now, what do we do? Our children are grown and middle-aged, many of our grandchildren are teenagers or young adults, some of us have great-grandchildren, we have retired or soon will be, and our "honey" have passed or are sickly, gone away, or struggling with what to do in their retirement. Fortunately, we have time, resources, and our "girlfriends" to support us.

The purpose is to record how you and your life have changed, to get in touch with your feelings, to awaken lost interests, or to find new ones. Here are the three assignments:

1. Daily Journaling

There is nothing like it! Oprah swears by it; Melodie Beatty (self-help guru and author on codependent relationships) preaches it; Sarah Ban Breathnach (her books, such as *Simple Abundance: A Daybook of Comfort and Joy,* have sold millions of copies) expounds on it; Julia Cameron (best known for her book, *The Artist's Way,*) insists on it! And Elizabeth J. Wheeler says, "Just do it!" Journal, baby! Nothing has given me more peace of mind and direction than writing each morning.

When you start your day, grab a notebook, and start writing. Be sure to include several specific things or situations you are grateful to have in your life. For example, write how you are feeling, what you are looking forward to, what you are scared of, who you are mad at, and what you don't know what to do about.

2. Weekly Outing

One day each week, go on a fun excursion. (Julie Cameron calls this an Artist Date, and she insists on it) It doesn't have to cost money unless you want to spend money on something special. The time I spend each week invigorates me, fertilizes my creativity, and puts me in touch with a source much more powerful than me. Here are some ideas: Go to a shop or restaurant you have always wanted to visit; take in a movie; go to another town and walk around; visit a playground or dog park; get a facial; or try on wigs.

In this space or your notebook, record the dates and places of your outings and any thoughts or feelings you had about them:

____

____

____

____

____

____

____

____

____

____

____

____

____

____

____

____

3. Review Your Life

This exercise is an expedition to find buried dreams and ideas like a treasure hunt.

Look at how your life had changed from when you were a little girl to now as a lady of a certain age. Then, write brief answers to these questions every ten years of your life.

A. Where did you live?

0-10____

10-20____

20-30 ____

30-40 ____

40-50 ____

50-60____

60-70 ____

70 and beyond____________________________________

B. Who lived with you?

0-10 ____

10-20 ____

20-30 ____

30-40 ____

40-50 ____

50-60 ____

60-70 ____

70 and beyond____________________________________

C. Where did you go to school?

 0-10 ____

10-20 ____

20-30 ____

30-40 ____

40-50 ____

50-60 ____

60-70 ____

70 and beyond_______________________________________

D. What were your academic achievements?

 0-10 ____

10-20 ____

20-30 ____

30-40 ____

40-50 ____

50-60 ____

60-70 ____

70 and beyond_______________________________________

 E. What sports did you play?

 0-10____

10-20 ____

20-30 ____

30-40 ____

50-60 ____

60-70 ____

70 and beyond_______________________________________

F. What did you do for fun?

0-10 ____

10-20 ____

20-30 ____

30-40 ____

40-50 ____

50-60 ____

60-70 ____

70 and beyond____

G. What "technology" did you use?

0-10 ____

10-20 ____

20-30 ____

30-40 ____

40-50 ____

50-60 ____

60-70 ____

70 and beyond ____

H. Where did you work?

0-10 ____

10-20____

20-30____

30-40____

40-50____

50-60____

60-70____

70 and beyond____

I. Who did you work for/with?

 0-10 ____

10-20____

20-30____

30-40____

40-50____

50-60____

60-70____

70 and beyond_______________________________________

J. What did you look like—what did you wear/hair?

 0-10 ____

10-20____

20-30____

30-40____

40-50____

50-60____

60-70 ____

70 and beyond_______________________________________

K. Who were your best girlfriends?

 0-10 ____

10-20 ____

20-30 ____

30-40 ____

40-50 ____

50-60 ____

60-70____

70 and beyond ______________________________________

Chapter 2

WHAT LIES AHEAD

"I Did It My Way"

Elvis Presley and Other Performers

In this chapter, we will get out our crystal ball and make educated guesses about our lives. Similar to what we did in the third homework assignment in the previous chapter, we will draw another chart and fill in the blanks. However, since the questions are in the future tense, we will write in our best-educated guesses. There are four age columns: 60-70, 70-80, 80-90, and 90 and beyond. Nationally known educator and writer Elinor Miller Greenberg calls this age range the final third of life.

She discusses rejuvenation and uses other "R" words, such as reinvention, redefinition, and resurgence. The title of the book she wrote with Fay Wadsworth Whitney, *A Time of Our Own*, succinctly defines this period of life because we no longer have the responsibilities we carried in our younger years.

This chapter will cover five topics:

1) Society's general belief about older women.

2) Starting the final third of life.

3) Personal changes in the coming years.

4) Techniques to dissipate fear.

5) It's your choice—as always! Take what you like and leave the rest.

<u>**Society's general belief about older women**</u>

It is important to note that American society's general belief is that this final bit of life is when women shrivel up and fade away. "Grandma stays home all day, watches television, complains about aches and pains, and eats cereal." That might be true for some women but not all. Many women find this time in their life the most active and creative period because they do not have the responsibilities inherent in other life phases.   Good ol' Grandma Moses, Anna Mary Robertson Moses, is often referred to as the perfect example of one who explored her creativity as a lady of a certain age and began painting in earnest at age 78.

For older women, part of becoming invisible in our society is the insidious actions of younger people who seemingly want to put us in our place as feeble elderly females. Decisions are automatically rendered, such as "Oh, she can't eat that because _______, or she's had a knee replacement or a heart attack." Their older companion or family member inevitably cringes and then gives in. Then, without asking the older woman what she prefers, the younger person takes control in an attempt to diminish.

This is a response that is not easy to say, "Thank you. I can take care of myself and don't need to be monitored. It will only make me weaker. If I need help, I will ask." But, it is common for the older woman to grin and bear it. Be nice. Soon, we give up, and our life is not our own, and what is the purpose of that?

It is a different situation if the other person asks first to be of help because it is not assumed the older woman can't take care of herself, and she doesn't feel demeaned if her response is, "Yes, please."

However, sometimes playing the little old granny card around abusive or degrading people is wise. You are aware of the situation and consciously choose how to handle it.

Starting the final third of life

When this stage of our life starts, being tired, not knowing what to do, and feeling blah are common feelings. Author Melody Beattie calls times like these "the in-between places or the void." It is an uncomfortable place because one part of our life stops or changes dramatically, and we don't know what to do now. She talks about appreciating these times in our lives because they eventually will illuminate the clues to the path ahead. So many times in my life, I found her explanation of this time was just what I needed because I thought something was wrong with me. I understand now that these periods allow me to rejuvenate, just like my garden soil does each winter.

It is so tempting when we are in this gray zone to get busy: play golf daily, sign up for every volunteer opportunity that comes our way, babysit grandchildren night and day, etc. It is tempting because this busyness keeps us from experiencing this uncomfortable situation. Sitting in this place with these feelings is not pleasant. But magically, the sun comes up, and suddenly you know you are ready to grow. There is a trail ahead that seems so alluring. It calls your name, and you know it is where you need to go.

Looking at the final third of life can be depressing. But instead of putting our heads in the sand and accepting our fate, we can identify what probably lies ahead and make prudent decisions, to make the best of it. And, looking at the final third of life can be so enlivening. We can genuinely dream and decide what to do to make it all come true.

<u>Personal changes in the coming years</u>

There will be physical, financial, relationship, and mental changes in the coming years. This book does not profess any specific course of action. Instead, each woman is encouraged to do research and make up her mind about what is best for her. Just because the doctor says, just because my husband says, just because my daughter says, or just because you-name-it says, is no reason any lady of a certain age has to do what she is told to or ought to do.

Our physical condition will change as we age. Dr. Atul Gawande, in his best-selling book, *Being Mortal: What Matters in the End*, states these physical changes are likely to occur: pelvic organ prolapse, the body's ability to regulate temperature deteriorates, sluggish circulation, slower metabolism, aging and drooping skin, insomnia, enamel wearing away from teeth, hearing loss, arthritis, tremors, small strokes, bones soften, blood vessels, joint, muscle, heart valves, lungs stiffen, and this is my favorite one—brain rattles inside the skull.

The financial situation often changes because of less income and more medical expenses.

Our relationships sometimes alter because our spouse dies or we divorce. There has been a dramatic divorce increase in older adults, both for first-time marriages and even higher for second-time marriages. Children have left the nest and have lives of their own. Estranged adult children are not uncommon.

Depression and addiction rates increase in older adults. According to the National Institute on Drug Abuse, substance abuse, and alcoholism rise dramatically for this age group.

The routine of daily life changes. Where once we might have greeted the receptionist at work each morning, now we say hello to our pets, yoga teacher, friends in our knitting group, or fellow members of a Zoom meeting. Homework assignment No. 5, the Anchors in Life Circle, shows many new relationships beyond our family. Our social network of girlfriends is paramount because they have similar experiences and give us support. Other significant groups often include religious, medical, and therapeutic organizations, household help, and pets.

<u>**Techniques to dissipate fear**</u>

Undoubtedly, fear and resentment will fly into our thoughts like mosquitoes bombarding our skin on a summer evening. Suddenly doubts about the future, our health, our family, financial concerns, etc., will bite us, so to speak. Identifying the worry by clearly defining it on paper can help us understand how it emotionally affects us socially, economically, or as older women. Then, to clarify what we might or might not do about the situation, we can ask ourselves several questions.

Here is the sequence of questions I used to help me:

- I'm fearful of?

- Why do I have this fear?

- How does this fear affect my self-esteem?

- How does this fear affect my personal relations?

- What are my hopes or ambitions about this situation?

- Where might I cause harm to myself or others?"

- What can I do differently?

- What is the worst that can happen?

- What do I gain from this, my pay-off, so to speak?

- What can I do to protect myself?

It's your choice—as always! Take what you like and leave the rest.

First and foremost, it is your choice and only yours as to what you want to do with your life. My purpose is to write about the topic of ladies of a certain age in a society that has ignored us. I present you with ideas based on research or personal experience. You can decide if my writing is relevant or valuable to you. I have stated from that very first blog I wrote that I wouldn't say I liked becoming invisible after a certain age; call it arrogant if you want, but I think who I was up to that point and what I had done mattered even if I was becoming wrinkled and gray-haired. I would be honored if you called me a feminist, but that is not what I set out to do. Fifty years ago, I was too busy having children, being a "corporate wife," and going to graduate school to engage in anything to promote women's rights. I just wanted to do certain things, even though back in the 1970s, those jobs would have been listed in the "Help Wanted–Men" section of the Sunday paper. Frankly, I never burned my bra and did not start marching until a couple of years ago when the thought of putting migrant kids in cages was just so disgusting to me. Nor did I like, once again, how women were being treated. So I joined the Women's March and many demonstrations since then.

So, if you choose to go down the traditional path of an older woman in America, that's your right. But our country needs older women more than ever before. We need their wisdom and accumulated knowledge. There is much-unfinished business from the 1970s, even though younger women have reaped the benefits of those times. I think more than ever before; we need to work together, whether we are 13, like my granddaughter, or 49, like her mom, or 74, like me, or my hiking buddy, soon to turn 80. But, of course, men (I'd say mostly older and white) are pushing back. After all, our behavior now is not what they are accustomed to, and we might do the job more effectively and efficiently and– hopefully, someday–at the same amount of pay.

These exercises aim to recognize feelings and interests and consider what you expected at this stage of your life and what might lie ahead. Here are the six assignments:

1. Daily Journaling

Writing will help you identify emotions that may be coming up now

2. Weekly Outing

Maybe you'll find your passion

3. Write two essays–as brief or as long as you like

Entitle the first essay, "What I expected my life to be like at this age."

Then write a second essay, "What is my life like now?"

They can be as brief or as long as you like.

4. Fill in this chart with what you expect to happen in the coming years for each area of your life

Area of Life	60-70	70-80	80-90	90 +
Family				
Health				
Wealth				
Work				
Relations				
Housing				
Dreams				
Travel				
Sports				
Hobbies				

After you finish this book, return to this chart and see if your expectations have changed.

5. Anchors in Life Circle

Draw a circle. Then draw four concentric circles around this first circle.

In the first circle, write your name.

In the second circle, write the name of your spouse or significant other if you have one.

In the third circle, write the names of your family members.

In the fourth circle, write the names of your friends.

In the fifth circle, write the names of people who provide essential services to you, such as your hairstylist, nail specialist, handyman, lawn mower, etc.

If appropriate, add more circles for coworkers, ministerial (church), therapeutic (medical and behavioral health), pet support, etc., and fill in the names.

As we go through life, the names in the circles change. I always thought that few things and people would change once I got to the latter third of my life. My expectation is invalid because life is not static. People come, go, die, grow away from each other, move, etc.

The people in the fifth circle become essential to us in the latter third of life. Reasons for this include: Number of single female heads of households, which increases as we age; families live in different geographic areas, and friends may move, become ill, die, or pursue other interests.

6. The put-the-old-lady-in-her-place exercise

Become aware of when someone is diminishing you. Then, as soon as practical, jot down the incident in your journal or notebook. Look for phrases such as "young lady" and "Oh, let me get that for you." Come up with responses. I came up with these two: "Well, actually, I haven't been a young lady for decades, but I am a proud 70-year-old," and "That's kind of you, but I prefer to do it myself."

Chapter Three

DEALING WITH HEALTH CHANGES

You put your whole self in,

You put your whole self out;

You put your whole self in,

And you shake it all about.

You do the Hokey-Pokey,

And you turn yourself around.

That's what it's all about

Disclaimer

I no longer serve as a spokesperson for any healthcare organizations I have worked for. Sources for this information are referred to and listed in the Resource section. It is not medical advice.

<u>This chapter will cover these six topics:</u>

1) Death and life.

2) Exercise.

3) Massage.

4) Diet.

5) Meditation.

6) Health–from your head to your toes.

This chapter focuses on the above topics because physical, mental, emotional, and spiritual concerns are intrinsically connected. It covers physical topics, starting with the head and ending with the toes, behavior, and emotional health, and emphasizes the immense importance of exercise, diet, and individual spiritual practice.

It does not go into drugs, procedures, or "recommended guidelines." Before you commit to taking medications or undergoing any procedures, I suggest you diligently research the topics and talk to women who have chosen them. "Recommended guidelines" are just that: recommended. Before you proceed, you might ask yourself, at my age, what the risk is versus the benefits. You do not immediately have to consent to these options, no matter how much pressure you get from healthcare professionals, family, or friends. The big takeaway is to consider your choices and healthcare and then decide what is best for you.

This personal approach to health is likely to be awkward for the ladies of a certain age in the first group of the Boomer generation. Remember, I call women born in the Boomer years Boomer Babes. There are two distinct groups: those born from 1946-1954 and those between 1955-1964. The second group sees the world very differently from the first group because of the rapid socioeconomic and technological changes in the United States following World War II.

Taught to respect authority, or you could say, "follow orders," the first group of Boomer Babes, those born between 1946-1954, is unlikely to question doctors or almost anyone in the medical profession since the country had just come out of the war.

When Boomer Babes in the second group (1955-1964) came along, society started questioning authority. To give a quick visual of the rapid changes in societal norms that took place from 1946 to 1964, I suggest you summon up the image of Elvis on the 1956 Sunday night CBS Ed Sullivan Show, which only showed the King of Rock and Roll from the waist up because of the country's sexual concern of his rotating hips. The country had "adjusted" to Elvis and his gyrations by the decade's end. But by the time 1964 rolled around, "those British guys with the long hair," the Beatles, rocked American sensibilities again on the popular entertainer's variety show. The Fab Four, as the Beatles were referred to, had just hit the top of the American charts for the first time with their song, "I Want to Hold Your Hand."

At first, taking care of our health seems simple at this age. After all, we have been taking care of ourselves for decades. But, as surgeon Atul Gawande, MD, in his New York Times No.1 bestselling book, *Being Mortal: Medicine and What Matters in the End,* states, "Our bodies do eventually wear out."

This information can scare the bejeebers out of you. And if that is not enough, pharmaceutical companies' advertisements vividly describe deteriorating or diseased bodily functions with paid actors!

Ladies of a certain age are constantly bombarded with health messages.

Where do we, as ladies of a certain age, start to choose how to deal with our health issues?

I suggest we first consider how we want to die.

Death and life

This suggestion might seem outrageous to you. Let me tell you a little personal experience that showed me how logical and practical this idea is. In April of 1986, my 68-year-old father told me his cancer had returned, and he was terminal. On August 6, he died. He spent the last four months of his life in a hospital, underwent many procedures, and took lots of drugs. He and his wife made those choices based on his doctors' recommendations. They did not ask my sister or me how we felt about these decisions. Even today, I feel cheated. I did not get to spend quality time with my father because of his operations, drug procedures, physical therapy sessions, and drug-induced unconsciousness. These procedures did not extend his life or enhance his well-being. But, he and his wife "followed doctors' orders." They never questioned or considered his quality of life or the time the doctors' orders took away from spending quality time with his family and loved ones.

Even with my father's excellent health insurance, this care cost thousands and thousands of dollars. His estate could afford these costs, but I have often thought what a waste of money for someone who was terminally ill, had a wife, two adult daughters, grandchildren, and many friends and associates who loved and respected him. Dad was just too busy and exhausted with medical interventions to spend time with us. I know he would have preferred that this money go to charitable organizations.

That experience—far more than the years I spent in healthcare marketing—has guided my choices on how I deal with aging and dying. Yes, I have a living will and advanced directives, and I have talked many times with my family about them. The importance of these documents is covered later in the chapter.

Dr. Gawande's book, *"Being Mortal: Medicine and What Matters in the End,"* solidified my thinking and feelings on these issues. It is my number one healthcare book recommendation.

So death is where this chapter begins. And to start, we must circle around to search our souls and ask ourselves how we want to live.

Here are some questions:

1. As we age, the probability of severe injuries from falls and chronic illnesses increases. We are besieged with this information by advertisers selling various products and services. Consequently, it is common for ladies of a certain age to restrict activities and focus on what might happen. Another choice, however, is to evaluate our environment for safety concerns and identify areas where we could make adjustments to continue to live the way we want to. Which do you prefer?

2. Have you talked with your family and/or significant others about how you want to live as a lady of a certain age? Do you want them to "check on you" regularly? Help you with all sorts of things in the house? Buy various technology things and set them up for you. Do you want them to be available to you if you need them? Do you want them not to tell you what to do? Do they know your daily routine and what is important to you? You may or may not want to do any of this.

Then, we must circle around to search our souls and ask ourselves how we want to die. Here are some questions to consider.

1) Do you want to prolong your life as long as possible with experimental drugs, chemotherapy, radiation, the use of a ventilator, or surgeries?

2) How do you want pain managed?

3) Where do you want to die?

4) Who, if anyone, do you wish to have with you at the end?

Discussing your wishes with family and or significant others can be awkward. It is not uncommon for people to avoid or forgo talking about "such things" while alive and well. These discussions are often hard but are more difficult and sometimes impossible when death is at the door. You may want to talk further if you and your loved ones have differing opinions. Ask them to read Dr. Gawande's book or bring in "experts" for more information. Consider bringing in a clergy member or a therapist into the discussion.

Now is the time to secure medical documentation to solidify your wishes and give direction to caregivers and medical professionals. Although these documents, medical power of attorney, living will, and an advanced directive sound very legal and possibly very expensive, they are essential if you want your care and your death to go (as much as possible) as you wish. The good news is that they do not need to cost you anything. Forms and information are readily available on the Internet. AARP's Amanda Singleton states, "Clear, written health care direction is a gift to those who love you."

A medical power of attorney is a designation that clearly states you have chosen the person named to make medical decisions when you no longer have the capacity to do so. For example, you may need your designee temporarily or for navigating a long-term health crisis.

Living wills, which are advanced directives and other directives, are written legal instructions regarding your medical care preferences if you cannot make decisions for yourself.

Of course, you will want to make sure that whomever you designate to be your medical power of attorney agrees with your wishes. This person does not have to be a family member.

Put a notarized durable medical power of attorney card in your wallet. Also, enter the names of your emergency contacts and the durable medical power of attorney information into your phone.

<u>Exercise</u>

The importance of daily exercise has been a hard concept for American ladies of a certain age to grasp, let alone accept. Major healthcare organizations such as The American Heart Association, The American Cancer Society, and Alzheimer's Association have published numerous studies that state the significance of exercise.

But, if it has not been part of your life in the past, exercise is a hard thing to start, to get into, and to make it an essential part of each day.

What I tell myself is, "Just do it and no excuses. Start slow and easy." It's impressive that you don't have to do anything extreme to gain immense benefits from exercise. Yoga, stretching, walking, and strength training daily improve health and mood.

"Just do it and no excuses" may sound dictatorial, and it doesn't get at the immense effort to change lifelong habits. I found this quote in *Meditations from the Mat: Daily Reflections on the Path of Yoga* by Rolf Gates and Katrina Kenison to be a softer, more comfortable, and maybe more effective approach. "If you are new to yoga, chances are you are wrestling not only with the postures but also with the judgments you pronounce on your efforts. But if you can commit to being a little easier on yourself, I am certain you will enjoy your practice more. If not, you may soon find yourself making all sorts of excuses to avoid practicing all together—it will become just too painful. When we opt out of experiences that challenge us, it's usually because our pride is in the way. And "pride" is another word for fear—the fear of not being enough."

Another challenge with exercise is which exercise is best for you. Like many women, I have found yoga to be beneficial. It has been the choice of many people for thousands of years. You can take yoga classes in person, at community, recreation, or fitness centers, or in the comfort of your own home via Zoom and YouTube. Some classes are free, some aren't, and the cost varies greatly.

Here are some items to consider:

1. There are many different types of yoga. The words can be very confusing. See the Resource section for an article about common styles.

2. Alignment is essential so that you do not injure yourself. Careful guidance from an instructor who gives you personal adjustments is critical.

3. Yoga, slowly paced, with lots of props for back, knees, shoulders, and feet issues, helps to ensure the most benefit of this practice.

4. Training for yoga instructors varies from a few weeks to many years. The more training your instructor has, the better that person is in a position to help you.

5. Instructors can be of any age or sex. An instructor you feel comfortable working with is the best.

6. Stretching keeps muscles long, lean, and supple, and it is part of the curriculum for yoga classes and many exercise programs for older people.

Perhaps, the queen of stretching is Canadian Miranda Esmonde-White, born in 1949. Her PBS show, "Classical Stretch," has been on television since 1999, and her *Eccentrics* classes are taught at many recreation and community centers and available online.

For most, walking is the easiest of all exercises. The key is to walk daily for approximately 30 minutes each time. An excellent prop to keep you on task and schedule is a dog. It is essential to have a well-trained dog so you walk the dog, and the dog doesn't walk you. This training is useful when you encounter a stray dog or one whose owner has no control over it. Be careful of retractable leashes. If your dog charges after something, the leash can pull your shoulder out. In bad or icy weather, community and recreation centers or shopping centers are safe walking places.

A little strength training each day goes a long way. Muscles start to decline after age 30, and bones weaken. Recreation, fitness, and community centers generally offer strength training for older people, and there are many YouTube videos available online.

For me, a simple 15-minute workout at home includes squats (back against the wall), sit-ups, lunges, leg step-ups, and arm workouts with light weights. I have found some good old rock 'n' roll music helps me get through this strength training exercise. It was amazing how weak my legs got after I moved from a two-story into a one-level house.

Massage

As we age, we often have fewer opportunities to be touched by a caring person. Yet, since the beginning of time, this simple gesture conveys caring and promoted healing.

Research has revealed the importance of touching as we age in the past couple of decades. Even massaging our skin helps our well-being.

The cover of the December 2015/January 2016 issue of *The AARP Magazine* promotes a feature article, "The Amazing Power of Touch," with a description "Heal your pain, lift your mood, skip the meds." Author Tiffany Field states, "… it increases activity along the vagus nerve that runs from the brain stem to the abdomen. Stimulating it can offer various benefits throughout the body, from improved digestion to a jolt of the mood-boosting neurotransmitter serotonin. It's the body's natural antidepressant."

In Dr. Christiane Northrup's book *Goddesses Never Age*, she has a whole section explaining the benefits of touch and massage. The famed doctor even writes, "In fact, I think massage should be a cornerstone of your self-care and wellness program."

A monthly massage may be an added expense to your budget but with a considerable return on investment.

Diet

So much has been written about this subject; I am going to synthesize the information with this simple list:

1. Don't eat junk food such as sugary processed cereals, chips, soda and snacks, hamburgers, fries, and milkshakes from fast-food chains.

2. Eat a minimum of five fruits and vegetables each day.

3. Protein is essential. Good sources include nuts, grains, eggs, beans, cheese, dairy, oats, quinoa, and guava. According to *Prevention Magazine,* people aged 65 and older need more protein. You do not need meat and fish to meet these needs unless you want to consume them.

4.   I believe in eating only organic fruit and vegetables. The additional cost is well worth not putting various chemicals in your body.

5. Grain: for example, oats, 100 percent whole wheat, kamut, and millet.

Fixing meals and eating alone can be difficult. Planning or finding new recipes, particularly ones for small serving sizes, can increase interest in eating and food preparation.

A dark green salad with a vinaigrette dressing is a great way of adding greens and veggies to your diet. Also, it can provide a protein source if nuts, cheese, etc., are added.

An easy way to check if you are getting balanced daily nutrition is to make sure you have eaten at each meal a vegetable and or fruit, a grain, and a protein source.

Personal note: I have found daily consumption of dark chocolate, coffee, and red wine essential for my health.

<u>Meditation</u>

People of all ages benefit from meditation, but the payback for ladies of a certain age is enormous, according to articles published by AARP and such prestigious publications as *U.S. News & World Report* (see Resources). The benefits include:

- Lowered breathing, heart, and blood pressure rates

- Improved digestion

- Sharpened and focused mind

- Reduced anxiety

- Increased relaxation

- Better management of moods and emotions

Many ladies of a certain age experience loneliness, sadness, and depression from the loss of significant people and pets and their independence at this stage of life. Daily meditation can help manage these feelings.

Like exercise, the critical consideration is the same for meditation–do it and make no excuses. Any form of meditation or style will work. You get to choose what is best for you.

Personal note: I have a simple meditation form that has worked for me for years. Each morning I sit on my living room couch, look out the front window and set a timer for 15 minutes. Then, I say a few special prayers, close my eyes, and listen for any sounds I hear. No, I have never gone to nirvana, but I always experience peace and gained knowledge about problematic areas in my life.

Health–From Your Head to Your Toes

This section will give you a concise rundown of some things you might experience. Even though I was in healthcare communications for decades, I was unaware of many of these health issues. One note: Financial planners explicitly say healthcare costs, including dental expenses, are drains on retirement budgets that many people don't anticipate.

Head

<u>Late-onset addiction to alcohol</u>

Wow, few want to discuss this big elephant in the living room. Widely reported are opioids and benzodiazepine addiction. However, good-old alcoholism in later life is a real shocker to many people. According to Sally K. Rigler, MD, of the University of Kansas School of Medicine, "One-third of older alcoholic persons develop a problem with alcohol in later life, while the other two-thirds grow older with the medical and psychosocial sequelae of early-onset alcoholism. Potential triggers include boredom in retirement, loss of income, death of loved ones, and decreased physical abilities."

<u>Cognitive and mental health concerns</u>

These include anxiety, sleep problems, depression, dementia, and Alzheimer's.

<u>Suicide</u>

Older adults experience one of the highest suicide rates of any age group, according to the American Foundation for Suicide Prevention.

Eyes

A yearly eye exam is a great insurance for dealing with these three common vision problems as we age: 1. Age-related macular degeneration (AMD) 2. Glaucoma, and 3. Cataracts. Early intervention may help with the first two, and cataract surgery can improve vision dramatically. Check with your doctor's office regarding Medicare and supplemental insurance coverage for eye exams and conditions.

Ears

Hearing loss is common. It can lead to not being able to hear essential sounds in life as well as isolation. Hearing aids and other devices have improved over the years, for example, rechargeable batteries and cell phone sound adjustment options. If you buy your hearing aids in one town and then move, hearing centers in the new location may not service your hearing aids or do so with significant charges.

Teeth

Routine dental exams are great insurance for dealing with the four most common dental problems for ladies of a certain age:

- Gum and periodontal disease

- Tooth decay

- Shrinking of gums

- Dry mouth

Seeing a dentist at least twice yearly for examination and cleaning, reasonable daily dental care, drinking plenty of water, and avoiding sugary foods and drinks can help you save your teeth and improve your health. Dental problems can lead to serious health problems throughout your body.

The Harvard Health Letter, "The Aging Mouth," published by the Harvard Medical School in 2010, states, "The well-being of your aging mouth is tied to the health of the rest of your body." Medical research suggests an association between gum inflammation and many aging-related diseases, such as heart disease, stroke, respiratory problems, and diabetes.

Gum and periodontal disease can slowly occur and not cause pain. Gum recession exposes softer root tissue of teeth, which leads to cavities, tooth loss, and health issues. It is treatable.

As the enamel on teeth weakens and biting edges are worn down, tooth decay increases. According to the Harvard Health Letter, "The rate of tooth decay in people over 65 now outpaces that of schoolchildren." Further, silver fillings from childhood or adolescence eventually break down. Also, decay can develop along the edges of these fillings.

The incidence of oral cancer increases with age, tobacco use, and mouth sores. During a dental examination, the doctor looks for oral cancer. A white or red patch in your mouth, tongue, or lips that lasts more than two weeks may be a sign of oral cancer and should be evaluated by a dentist.

A dry mouth raises the risk of gum disease and tooth decay. It can be caused by medications, alcohol, caffeinated beverages, tobacco, and decreased saliva production because of aging. Drinking more water is essential for a variety of health reasons for older adults.

Medicare does not cover most dental work, which often is quite expensive. It is astute planning to save for these costs and to consider a supplemental plan.

Dehydration

According to the Cleveland Clinic's 2018 article, "Drink Up: Dehydration is an Often Overlooked Health Risk for Seniors," older people frequently do not feel thirsty and have reduced awareness of body temperature. Further, the body's water content decreases with aging. Besides causing dental problems, dehydration can lead to fainting, confusion, dizziness, muscle cramps, and strength loss.

Skin

Any lady of a certain age will tell you she does not feel invisible by the skin and face beauty products industry!

Our skin ages. Dark spots, wrinkles, pre-cancerous growths, skin cancer, and dry and itchy patches are just a few of the conditions experienced. To check for skin cancers, consider a yearly skin screening by a dermatologist.

Then there are the numerous and various claims for cosmetics and skincare products. Like lipstick, cream, and foundation, many of these products contain petroleum byproducts, injurious to health. I have included information for you to review in the homework area. Keep a list of the most dangerous products. I have such a list on my phone and consult it before I buy products.

Bones and joints and all of our organs

Daily exercise and excellent nutrition are the measures to help with the predictable decline.

Pelvic organ prolapse

I don't remember this subject ever being discussed in health classes I took in school or birth preparation workshops.   It is somewhat embarrassing, but if you have had a baby through your vagina, you will likely have pelvic organ prolapse, which means some of your body tissue can stick out of your vagina. Other things can raise your risks, such as obesity, smoking, and constipation. In addition, it can lead to urinary or fecal incontinence, urinary tract infections, and painful sex.

Nonsurgical treatment is the use of a pessary. Inserted into the vagina is a rubber-like ring device. A gynecologist or pelvic health specialist can measure and fit the device. It has to be cleaned regularly and examined by a professional, generally every year. The best article I found on the subject, "What to do about pelvic organ prolapsed, was published by the Harvard Medical School. It is listed in the Resource section.

Feet

You will often hear in a yoga class, "We start with the feet because of the vast number of nerve endings, and imbalances in the feet can lead to ankle, knee, hip, and back problems."

As we age, bunions, falling arches, and in-grown toenails often are challenges. Feet exercises like yoga and other practices can help with bunions and falling arches. A monthly pedicure can keep ingrown toenails in check. Also, as we age, nails thicken, making it difficult to trim toenails.

The purpose is to understand how you want to live and die, explore the benefits of massage, yoga, and exercise, seek dental and eye care, understand health care, and discover harmful chemicals in beauty products. Here are nine assignments:

1. Describe the time in which you die. Who is with you? Where are you? What are you looking at? Do you smell anything? What are you wearing? What are you feeling?

2. Attend an advanced directives workshop or seminar. These are generally free and available in most communities.

3. Review the AARP website on advanced directives.

4. Get a massage.

5. Find out what yoga and exercise classes your community offers.

6. For a week, record what you eat and drink each day and the amount.

7. If you don't already have one, find a dentist you like and make an appointment.

8. If you don't already have one, find an eye doctor you like and schedule an appointment.

9. Research your health insurance coverage for dental and eyecare examinations and hearing aids

Chapter Four

WHERE DOES MONEY COME INTO ALL OF THIS?

Money don't get everything, it's true

What it don't get, I can't use

Now, give me money (That's what I want!)

The Beatles

I wish I could sugarcoat the importance of money for ladies of a certain age, but I can't. It would be very deceiving if I did. Frankly, ladies, this is where the rubber meets the road. And I hate to tell you that no financial advisor will save you by waving a magic wand. If managing money has not been your thing, well, now is the time to do so and stop pretending prince charming, something or somebody–God knows what–is going to save you.

For those of you with husbands or significant others, please note: If you haven't been involved in your finances, now is the time to do so. Ideally, both of you will be involved in planning your financial future.

If you think you can skip this chapter because your partner handles the finances, the stories of these women may change your mind. Each of the four women paid dearly for not participating in marital financial affairs: One woman lived in the height of luxury: she had a big house and yacht and wore designer clothing. One day her 60-something husband died, and she quickly learned they were hocked up to their ears. She had no idea of the financial situation and now lives in a studio apartment. A second woman did not know what retirement dollars she had to live on when her husband died, and his company pension quit coming in. Her standard of living dropped from comfortable to meager. A third woman never delved into the family finances because she did not want her husband to think she did not trust him. As a result, she had a rude awaking when he left her after 45 years of marriage. A fourth woman had an emotionally abusive relationship with her alcoholic husband. She feared his rage if she started to ask questions. She never knew until he died that many years earlier that she could have left the marriage financially comfortable.

If you want to be financially safe and secure in the latter third of life, Suze Orman–America's guru for women and finances, says, "You're never powerful in life until you're powerful over your own money".

If you have been managing your money all along and planning for retirement, chapter four will give you some pause and an opportunity to consider double-checking your efforts.

<u>This chapter covers these six topics:</u>

1) Identifying personal feelings and beliefs about money because they are the basis for all your financial decisions up until now.

2) Defining your principles, a personal foundation, for your financial decisions for the latter third of your life.

3) Listing your dreams for the future along with estimates of cost.

4) Outlining your financial goals.

5) Summarizing current and future sources of income and expenses.

6) Deciding if you need a financial advisor.

Two homework assignments and a list of resources in the appendix will assist you with this critical planning.

The first exercise, "Money Madness, " is beneficial before delving further into these six topics.

<u>Identifying personal feelings and beliefs about money because they are the basis for all your financial decisions up until now</u>

For many women, this is the key to financial success now and in the future because most people have no idea how feelings and beliefs impact their financial decisions. This introspection will take time and involve walking through your childhood and early adult years. You may or may not want to share this with others. Sometimes the revelations can be painful. You may even feel some shame. But, once you get them out, you will remove any sting that has been festering, maybe for years.

Begin by getting a notebook and daily setting time aside to do this. Yes, it is worth it. Start by listing each of your memories about money on a page, starting with the earliest ones. Here are some of the things I wrote down:

Age 4—my mother read me the fairytale "Little Match Girl."

Age 6—begging my mother to save StarKist Tuna labels and then mailing them to the company for an inflatable Charlie the Tuna so he and I could play in my little swimming pool in the backyard.

At 8—establishing a Christmas account at University Hills Bank to have money to buy my family Christmas presents. (I still remember what I bought them!)

Age 11—remembering my next-door neighbor and best friend getting her very own pink Princess phone in her room. (We had just gotten a second phone at our house. It was in my parent's bedroom.)

Age 14—earning $200, the cost of contact lenses, babysitting, mowing the family lawn, etc., because my dad told me if I wanted those "new-fangled contact things," I would have to pay for them.

Throughout my childhood and teen years, my mother's insistence that I stop sucking my thumb, turning in my foot, taking care of my skin, and watching my weight so I would become pretty (because, you know, that is how you got a man to marry you, build you a big house, and have lots of money.)

Next, under each memory, write down the answers to these five questions:

1. How did that memory affect my self-esteem? I felt great and powerful that I got Charlie the Tuna!

2. How did that memory affect my relations? I think my mom was pleased with my determination because she often told me that as a young girl, during the Depression, she would walk to the neighborhood store to ask the butcher for free bones for her dog. The bones were for her mom's soup. The family did not have any pets.

3. How did that memory affect my material security? I would get what I wanted if I convinced my mom to buy tuna and save the labels. No surprise, I later went into public relations!

4. How did this memory affect my emotional security? I felt confident I could get what I wanted by working with others and convincing them of my needs.

44

5. How did this memory affect my thoughts about being a girl?

Even back then, I thought if I were a boy, my mom would buy all the required number of tuna cans, take off the labels, and mail them in. Boys always got what they wanted, after all!

Now, write a sentence or two about what you learned about money based on the answers to the five questions for each memory. For example, I wrote this based on Charlie the Tuna:

If I worked hard enough and pleased others, I would get what I wanted.

It is important to note that we all have our own beliefs and feelings that influence our financial decisions and life decisions, for that matter. What I believed was very different from my sister's. Maybe because she never wanted Charlie the Tuna!

It is also important to note that once you have identified your feelings and beliefs, you can question them and decide if you still want them to influence your life.

Defining your principles, a personal foundation, for your financial decisions for the latter third of your life

Again, time spent on introspection will pay off in big bucks. Write down the answers to each of these questions:

1. How comfortable am I with debt?

2. How do I feel about risk?

3. Do I trust people to help me with money?

4. Must I now provide a financial safety net for my children, grandchildren, or other family or friends?

5. Should I leave something for them when I die?

6. Is it more important to travel or to have financial security?

7. Am I concerned about who will care for me personally and financially if I get sick?

8. How much time do I want to spend managing and accounting for my money?

List personal principles for your future financial foundation.

These three principles anchor my foundation: One, I wanted to live within my means. Two, I would adjust my lifestyle to do so. Three, I would find and use a simple method to track money.

List your dreams for the future, along with estimates of the cost.

Now is the time to list dreams for the future and estimate their associated costs. These dreams will become the motivators for achieving the goals you set to obtain them.

You may already have a list of dreams, a bucket list, if you will, for what you want to do in the latter third of your life, or perhaps, you don't and need to figure out what you want to do.

If you already know what you want to do, write it down, or put it in black and white, as they say. There is something about writing that helps us identify and achieve our goals. Take a look at your list. Ask yourself these questions: Is this what I want to do now that I think about it? Have I forgotten to jot something down? Are there other things I would like to do?

Now, put away your list for at least a week. When you pull it out again, ask yourself the same questions. Add or take off anything that strikes you.

Next, determine what you need to achieve your dreams regarding time, money, people, health, and other considerations. Write each of these down under the particular item. If you don't know an answer, research to find what you need.

If you don't know what you want to do or only have a few ideas, now is the time to start dreaming and researching. You can go to chapter six and read the whole section on bucket lists. I have found no better way to do this than to go through Julia Cameron's book, *The Artist Way*. Whether you view yourself as an artist or not, her information and tools have been invaluable to thousands. Additionally, you can review many websites that can help manufacture a bucket list and various books and classes to explore.

Some of my dreams included travel, playing various sports, and moving to Colorado's Western Slope. I wanted to go to every country where my ancestry had immigrated and take each of my three grandchildren to Europe. One of my dreams was to play specific golf courses, backcountry skiing, and snowshoeing as much as possible. I had lived in Grand Junction during the 1980s and loved it. My dream was to live there permanently someday.

Oh ***someday!*** I learned a harsh lesson one sunny hot day listening to the radio in my kitchen. I heard the famous Royal Gorge Carousel in southern Colorado was burning in a terrific fire. I started to cry. I had so wanted to see it. What I learned that day was not to put off your dreams.

Now is the time to list them and determine what it will take to achieve them. These actions and accomplishments motivate me going forward in the remaining years of my life.

Outlining your financial goals

Many have the goals listed below when they are considering retirement. Your goals may differ if your dreams are minimal or you have vast sums of money available. Regardless of your income, you must consider social security benefits and retirement income before developing your plans. Below are the goals I set for myself:

1. No house payment

2. No car payment

3. No debt

4. A nest egg, an emergency fund of three to six months of expenses in a bank savings account

5. A simple way to keep track of all monthly expenses

6. A realistic budget

From my experience, life is hard for women in the latter third of life who have not achieved these goals. Their life often includes living with family, subsidized housing, or housing that could be better. Many of them work either full or part-time. Some are bitter because their dreams are unlikely ever to come true. Unexpected health expenses become financially devastating.

One woman told me, "Elizabeth, tell your readers that not taking Social Security until age 70 or working full-time in some job past 70 is just not worth it. Our bodies wear down, and physically working that hard becomes very difficult."

If paying off your house or car is unrealistic for you before you retire, consider looking for housing you can afford after retirement and a vehicle that would meet your transportation needs. Then, sell your house while you are still working and move into what you can afford. Likewise, you can get out of your car payment now and get a vehicle you buy with cash.

<u>Summarize current and future income and expense sources.</u>

Since both income and expenses will change in the latter third of life, summarize them now and compare them to what you anticipate they will be. This is critical information as you enter the next phase in planning for future finances. If you still need to start using software to track income and expenses, consider getting something like Quicken and learning how to use it.

Here is a partial list:

- How much money do I have?

- Where is the money located? (bank accounts, etc.)

- How much money is coming in each month?

- How much money will go in when I retire?

- Do I have any credit card debt? If so, how much, and which cards?

- How much is my house payment or monthly rent?

- How much are my property taxes?

- How much do I pay for house insurance?

- How much are my homeowners' fees?

- How much do I pay for routine house maintenance?

- How much do yard and lawn care costs?

- Do I have a car payment or a car lease payment? If so, how much?

- How much do I pay yearly for heating and cooling my house?

- How much is my car insurance?

- How much do I pay for car license plates?

- How much money do I need for necessities?

- What does health insurance cost now?

- What will it cost in the future?

- Will my nest egg cover costs such as hearing aids and dental work?

- How much do I pay for cable?

- How much do I pay for phone service?

- How much do I pay for news services?

- Who does my yearly state and federal taxes, and how much does that cost?

- How much money do I donate every year, and to which organizations?

- How much money will I need monthly for my future dreams?

After you have everything listed, you can devise a budget for after you quit working based on a good idea of your monthly income and how much expense it will support. You should consider reducing your expenses and or eliminating some in the future. Consider small monthly fees because they can add up over time. Knowing how much they equate to over a year is a good idea.   Remember what Benjamin Franklin said, "Little strokes fell great oaks."

While still working, try living as you think you will in retirement. There is nothing like experience to shed light on the validity of plans.

Also, you will need a plan for organizing and tracking your retirement income and expenses.   For example, I arranged to have my retirement funds deposited automatically into my checking account. I set up another account to collect yearly income, such as my IRA distribution. I transfer monies from that account into checking when I need to.

Finally, besides being personally helpful, this information on income and expenses is essential for anyone trying to settle your estate, and letting that person know where to find it is the first step. The next step is keeping it updated.

Because I do not have a considerable estate as defined by my state, I decided to use Quicken WillMaker, an estate planning software, to establish my end-of-life legal documents.

Deciding if you need a financial advisor

A financial advisor can be vital if you need help managing your investments and creating a future financial plan. It is important to note that financial advisors are not fairy godmothers and that you, and you alone, have the responsibility to deal with your money.

If you already have a financial advisor that you are comfortable working with and are pleased with the service you are getting, this section might not help you. However, even if you are satisfied with the relationship, you may want to evaluate it and even interview other advisors now.

The most important considerations are the advisor's credentials, transparency in billing, and comfort with the personal relationship you have with that person.

A Certified Financial Planner (CFP) is a recognized standard in this field for expertise in financial planning, insurance, taxes, retirement, and estate planning. The Certified Financial Planner Board of Standards, Inc. awards the certificate to those who pass the CFP Board's exams and annual education programs.

The designation includes meeting formal education requirements, performance on the CFP exam, relevant work experience, and professional ethics. In addition, the recipient must have a bachelor's or higher degree from an accredited university or college recognized by the U.S. Department of Education and complete a list of specific financial planning courses.

If you are considering an advisor who does not have this designation, you will want to investigate their qualifications and knowledge. Ask how they make money and if you can talk with clients for references.

For all advisors, look up the person on the internet. Look for information on services, fees, total assets under management, investment companies, socially conscious funds, responsible investments they are associated with, client data, and location.

When you meet with the person in their office, review your surroundings. Try and get a sense of the office atmosphere. Ask yourself, is this a place I would like to work? No matter how high the individual is rated, look elsewhere if you have a bad feeling or are uncomfortable.

These questions may help: what investment strategy do they most often use in crafting clients' financial plans; what kind of clients do they typically work with; how many clients do they have that match your demographic; and what are their professional certifications and credentials?

Financial advisors generally make money in three ways:

1. Client fees, either hourly or percentage of assets under management

2. Commissions for certain financial transactions like securities and insurance products

3. Salaries if they are on the staff of a financial planning organization

A fee-only advisor does not get commissions. A fee-based advisor earns money from a combination of client fees and commissions.

Commissions can be a conflict of interest since the advisor's pay includes an incentive for the product sold.

According to Wikipedia, "A registered investment adviser (RIA) is a firm that is an investment adviser in the United States, registered as such with the Securities and Exchange Commission or a state's securities agency. The numerous references to RIAs within the Investment Advisers Act of 1940 popularized the term closely associated with the term *investment adviser*. The Securities and Exchange Commission defines an investment adviser as an individual or a firm that is in the business of advising about securities. However, an RIA is an actual firm, while the firm's employees are called Investment Adviser Representatives (IARs).

Registered investment adviser firms receive compensation through fees for financial advice and investment management. They are required to act as a fiduciary. This is very different from broker-dealers and their representatives, who provide recommendations for a commission. Broker-dealers and their representatives are not required to act as fiduciaries; they must make suitable recommendations for a client. This is a different standard of care, but most consumers need to be made aware of the difference, as any of these professionals may call themselves financial advisors.

In some instances, a firm may be "dual-registered," meaning they are a registered investment adviser along with being registered as a broker-dealer. In that case, they may provide advice for a fee and collect a commission on certain product sales.

Finally, reading financial publications will help determine if you need a financial advisor. Regardless, this will help you stay up to date on current issues. Here is a partial list of respected financial publications:

- *The Economist*

- *Kiplinger's*

- *Investor's Business Daily*

- *Bloomberg Business Week*

- *Barron's*

The purpose of this chapter's homework is to understand how you feel about money, to become aware of noted financial periodicals, and investigate financial management software. Here are three assignments:

1. Do the "Money Madness" exercise from Julia Cameron's book, *The Artist Way,* by completing the following phrases:

People with money are_____________________________________

Money makes people____

I'd have more money if_____________________________________

My dad thought money was__________________________________

My mom always thought money would ________________________

In my family, money caused ________________________________

Money equals ____

If I had money, I'd ______________________________________

If I could afford it, I'd_________________________________

If I had some money, I'd__________________________________

I'm afraid that if I had the money, I would ______________

Money is ____

Having money is not_______________________________________

Money causes ____

In order to have more money, I'd need to ________________

When I have money, I usually ____________________________

I think money ____

If I weren't so cheap, I'd ______________________________

People think money ______________________________________

Being broke tells me ____________________________________

2. Go to the library or your favorite bookstore and read several issues of *The Economist, Kiplinger's, Investor's Business Daily, Barron's,* and *Bloomberg Business Week.*

3. Investigate one or more software applications for financial management, such as Quicken.

Chapter Five –

A HOUSE FOR THE LATTER THIRD OF LIFE

"My house is me and I am it. My house is where I want to be and it looks like all of

my dreams."

Daniel Pinkwater

Not every woman moves after she retires, but many do. They want a smaller house with no stairs, or a location that doesn't require shoveling snow, or they want to be closer to grandkids, or their husbands want to… or, for many reasons.

Sometimes there are extenuating circumstances why women move later in life. For example, the need to move because of health concerns, the death of a spouse, divorce, economic reasons, the need to care for grandkids or elderly parents, etc.

Even if you plan not to move, you never know what's ahead in the latter third of life. This information may be very helpful to you.

<u>This chapter covers eight topics:</u>
1) Deciding where to start in your planning process.

2) Clearly and succinctly defining why you want to move.

3) Determining where you want to live.

4) Looking at different types of housing and associated costs.

5) Financing.

6) Selling your current home.

7) Moving process.

8) Establishing yourself in a new community.

<u>Deciding where to start in your planning process</u>

You may already know you want to move or should move. You may already know where you want to move to and what type of housing you want. You may not.

However, sometimes our conscious mind does not divulge our real needs and desires. Therefore, it's best to determine these before you go through "all the trouble of moving!"

Doing a little dreaming is an excellent place to begin the planning process. The first homework assignment could be beneficial before leveling into this chapter.

<u>Clearly and succinctly define why you want to move.</u>

Write this definition down. You can refer to it later when you are dead tired and the moving van is coming the next day. Your answer may include things like I want something other than a house payment. I don't want to pay all these taxes. I never want to shovel snow again. I want to live close to my kids. These stairs are killing me. I want a new house, an old one, or a different one. I want to be able to walk to the grocery store. I want to live in a college town so I can attend classes and presentations.

<u>Determining where you want to live</u>

You may already know. You may not. You may have a general idea. If you know where you want to live or have a general idea, spend some time in the location to see how it is. Visiting various sites might bring clarity if you don't know where you want to live. You may also want to contact groups you will likely join when you move. Meeting people with similar interests may help you decide if a specific community is for you. One woman told me she attended church services in different cities she was looking at and talked to members afterward.

Looking at different types of housing and associated costs

In days gone by, the selection was narrow. Now, there are a plethora of housing choices for seniors. Here are some options: Single-family homes, one-level homes, apartments, duplexes, condominiums, "lock-and-leave-community," retirement communities, 50-plus community, low-income apartments, alley houses, mobile homes, communal housing, extended care, and assisted living.

Each type of housing has its associated cost. The expenditure may include homeowners' association fees (monthly or yearly), property taxes, housing insurance, utilities, and maintenance. While these costs can be estimated, many others can't and can arise. A good house inspection may identify many of these, but not all.

Other costs may include closing, emergency repairs, home appraisal, inspection, loan origination fees, and mortgage interest.

Financing

Any mortgage on a house comes with the risk of not paying it off if you cannot maintain your income after retirement, and unforeseen expenses as you age could affect your ability to pay.

The ideal situation is to pay cash for a home and to have enough income for house and emergency expenses.

However, many people near retirement or those who have retired get mortgage loans. The Equal Credit Opportunity Act prohibits lenders from denying mortgages based on age. The key factor for lenders is the ability of borrowers to repay regardless of age.

In the latter third of life, borrowers must look at their ability to pay mortgages based on their current and, more importantly, future income. In addition, a sufficient cash reserve is necessary for emergency and unplanned expenses, such as medical and dental costs and other expenditures needed to maintain their home and life.

One way to avoid a mortgage is to sell your home and use some profit to pay cash for a smaller residence and invest or save the rest. Another strategy is to pay off all debt, including costly credit card debt. Living within one's means is key to having enough money to last throughout the latter third of life.

Another consideration to consider before applying for a mortgage is taxes. The 2019 tax reform bill increased the standard deduction. This bill eliminated one of the significant benefits of having a mortgage. Because of the deduction increase, fewer retired people itemize their taxes because their income needs to be higher to benefit from this new law. It did help people who have the income to benefit from itemized taxes.

If the new home needs improvements, such as high-impact glass used in hurricane-prone areas or heavy-duty air conditioners for hot locations, an estimate of cost before purchase is wise. Then consider how you would finance unless you plan on paying for the changes forthright. Home equity loans and mortgage refinancing are available to seniors. A home equity loan allows you to use the equity in your house to get immediate cash. When the loan is approved, fees and closing costs are required. If this loan becomes delinquent, the home could go into foreclosure.

Selling your current home

Here are some primary considerations:

- You will probably be shocked if you last bought or sold a house a little while ago. For one thing, most, if not all, of the process is electronic.

- Google zillow.com, realtor.com, and trulia.com, then type in your address. Each of these real estate sites will give you an estimated value for your home. This amount will provide you with a good idea of your sales price. Also, put in the addresses of houses near you similar to yours that have recently sold. This information will help clarify the asking price for your home, and the pictures will give you a good idea of the condition and appeal of these houses.

- Go to several open houses and see the condition of the homes for sale.

- Interview at least three real estate agents to determine if you can work with them, their commission fee (yes, it varies!), and their strategy for selling your home.

- Consider using a Senior Real Estate Specialist (SRES®). This is a designation awarded by the National Association of Realtors for training to deal with matters frequently associated with older buyers and sellers.

- Have an inspection done before you list your property. Yes, it will cost you money, but it will also tell you what repairs are needed. Best you find out now and fix the issue(s) before anything becomes a sticking point during the inspection process.

- Clean, clean, clean!

61

- It may be shocking when someone half your age, with different views on life and houses, tours your home.

Moving Process

Much depends on how far away you plan to move, your finances, and your physical and emotional health. If you use a moving company, get at least three estimates. Packing is very strenuous and can be expensive. Family and friends may be available to you, or you may need to hire someone. Boxes are often available in supermarkets, furniture, and liquor stores. Investigate the cost of various packing materials. If you are on Nextdoor.com, an internet site for neighborhoods nationwide, you may find moving boxes, often yours, for picking them up. Likewise, this site is an excellent way to eliminate the boxes after you move and unpack.

Establishing yourself in a new community

Because isolation can be very depressing for ladies of a certain age, establishing yourself in your new community is essential. Investigate and go to various functions. You don't have to commit to any of them. Start with a similar network you had, for example, your church, 12-step meeting, volunteer groups, fabric arts groups, library book clubs, etc. Many communities have newcomer groups and meet-up groups.

Homework assignments and a list of resources in the appendix will assist you with this critical planning.

Chapter five's homework aims to understand what you may like in a new home, where you would like to live and determine which of your possessions you would like to bring. Here are three assignments:

1. If you don't know where you want to move or what type of dwelling would be best for you, this exercise may help. Remember when you were a little girl, and you thought about what life was like if you were a princess, a movie star, a nurse, a doctor, a teacher, etc? Now, envision yourself in various roles for your latter third of life. Perhaps, you want to be a writer, an artist, a scratch golfer, a nonprofit leader, etc. Then, with each role, imagine where you would live. Write the various answers down in a notebook. Next, remember your bedroom as a child. What was it like? What did you like about the color of the walls, the windows, your bed, etc.? Write down what you remember in the same notebook. Finally, go to your library and see if they have a stack of old magazines you might have. Go through them and cut out any pictures of places that attract you. Glue them on a large poster board and put them in your office or wherever you have space.

I went through this process. It helped me clarify what I wanted and showed me how impractical some of my dreams were. I enjoy where I live now, and I love my house. Believe it or not, what I enjoyed most about my childhood bedroom, which I shared with my sister, were the corner windows. They let in so much light and a view of our neighbor's trees and rose garden. Well, guess what? My house now has big, tall windows with views of trees and rose gardens.

2. If you are still determining the geographic location you want to move to, jot down your top three choices and plan on spending several days or weeks in each. These trips may sound expensive, but they could save you the pain of relocating to the wrong area. While you are there, pretend you already live there. Try to stay close to a neighborhood that interests you. Envision an average day: Go to the grocery store, attend church, meetings you are interested in, see what the library system offers, investigate recreation and senior centers and museums, and look at hospitals and clinics, and universities and colleges.

3. Moving is expensive! Plan on spending several months before moving and going through each room of your house. Sell, donate, or give away anything that you do not want. Refrain from assuming your family will take your stuff. Ask them first. Go to consignment or thrift shops and see what is for sale and the costs of items. What you may think to be very valuable, say your china, may not be anymore. *Get The Life-Changing Magic of Tidying Up: The Japanese Are of Decluttering and Organizing*, by Marie Kondo.

Chapter Six –

WILL I HAVE A PURPOSE?

"Coming of age means

we can refuse to be confined to the kindly docile feathered grab

we're supposed to roost in."

Susan J. Douglas

Heck, yes, that is the answer! That is the reason I started writing so many years ago a monthly missive, a blog for those invisible, powerful, dynamic women ladies of a certain age.

And our purpose is more important than ever. The world needs us: bright, intelligent, wise women. We know the hypocrisy of marketers, particularly those selling beauty products and pharmaceuticals, which have ground into this country's very soul that older women have no value with their gray hair, wrinkles, and baggy skin. We are priceless, pure gold, and have much to contribute to this world.

This chapter covers these four topics:

    1)   Giving yourself time and tender loving care.

    2)   Just say, "Yes!"

    3)   Deciding what to do in the latter third of life.

    4)   Time management.

<u>Giving yourself time and TLC (tender loving care)</u>

"Inner time is especially needed at the beginning of a new season of your life," states author Jean Shenoda Bolan, M. D.

Time and TLC don't seem to go together for ladies of a certain age. After all, aren't women, especially older women, expected to give and give and give to their employers, spouses, children, families, community, and coworkers?

Time just for you? No way!

But time and tender loving care are precisely what women of a certain age need as they go through numerous transitions in the latter third of their lives. Slowing down and focusing on needs is essential when one way of life ends and another begins.

Yes, you will find your purpose, but first, you must enter this new life phase slowly, savoring each experience.

Stopping the ongoing busyness of routine life, hopping off the squirrel cage of activity, and resting —like 8 hours or more sleep every day— are the most important things to do now. Also, daily eating nutritious food and doing some exercise are critical. After all, we have been in high gear for decades and can now shift into a lower gear. Our bodies, minds, and souls need an adjustment period.

In good time we will come to know our future purpose in life. Trees know this. Every year they go dormant in the winter to rest; however, come the longer days of late winter and early spring, their sap once again begins to flow, and their buds soon swell.

"Take rest; a field that has rested gives a beautiful crop," stated Roman poet Ovid.

There's nothing wrong with getting into your pajamas early, drinking a warm cup of milk or cocoa, putting socks on your feet, and corralling a cuddly cat if that is your pleasure.

Massages, yoga classes, daily walks in nature, working in the garden, and playing with a silly dog are all activities that soothe the soul and nerves after decades of doing, doing, doing.

To gain a new perspective on life, get away from your environment on a personal retreat to a resort, campground, or cabin. A sojourn is extremely helpful for a shattered nervous system. It can even serve as a vision quest for what's next.

So just say, "Yes!"

It's one thing to take a little time off to rejuvenate; it's another to do nothing or stagnate. Watch out for isolation and your mind trying to justify its benefits. Isolation can lead to all sorts of physical and mental problems, addictions, and despair. It's doubtful you will find your purpose if you isolate.

A great way to figure out your "next chapter" is to say "yes" to invitations from families and friends, even if you don't want to. You never know; the new adventure might be the very activity that points you to your future path.

Also, "just say yes," even if the person asking is older or younger than you. Friends are so crucial to ladies of a certain age. They are our buffers to life, an asset to have in tough times and good times, and resources when we don't know the way.

Throughout the ages, women have worked together. They helped one another have babies, quilt, cook for the tribe, do PTA assignments, and implement neighborhood parties, stenographer pools, and corporate teams. Women covered "other women's backs." They talked about their problems, fears, joys, and challenges during their time together. Women are comparative by nature, not competitive like men. Friends become even more critical as we age and undergo many life changes and losses. Our children have left us and have their own families, many of our men have gone, and we no longer have our profession or work. Boomer men, on the other hand, often have difficulty adjusting to retirement. They do things with the boys but don't talk with them.

Mary, my mother-in-law, was one of my role models until her death at age 99! We remained friends after my divorce from her son. Her children lived far away from her small Minnesota town on the Canadian border. She might have completed the eighth grade. She was a widow for a good 20 years or so. "Quit dying my hair after Pa died and never baked another loaf of bread," she proudly told me. Mary had lots of younger friends. Some of them were my age or younger. They did many things together, including going to Canada to drink and gamble. Mary had a blast. Everyone knew Mary, and I did not know one person who did not think the world of her. Almost until her death, she gardened, proudly shoveled her walks, shared lots of baked goodies and donuts, and was a regular at the senior community center and her church.

Deciding what to do in the latter third of life

I'm pretty sure my mother-in-law did not devise a seven-point plan to discover her life's purpose in her older years. Recently, when the topic of strong women came up, my 50-year-old daughter said, "Yeah, Grandma could kick ass, too." She showed us how to enjoy life and how not to be negated by anyone. If she had a plan, I'm sure her number one goal would have been to have fun with her friends and to enjoy life.

It would be nice if we could go to Harry Potter's school, Hogwarts, and attend the sorting ceremony shortly after entering this period of our life. We would sit on a stool, and a big hat would hover over us and proclaim what we would do.

Oh, you may not think I'm pretty,

But don't judge on what you see,

I'll eat myself if you can find

A smarter hat than me.

You can keep our bowlers black,

Your top hats sleek and tall,

For I'm the Hogwarts Sorting Hat

And I can cap them all.

There's nothing hidden in our head

The sorting Hat can't see,

So try me on and I will tell you

Where you ought to be.

From *The Sorcerer's Stone*, by J.K. Rowling

You know the clichés: Time marches by, blink, and it is gone, time is of the essence, and no one is guaranteed tomorrow. But, as tired as these phrases sound, time will just zoom by without planning what you want to do during this precious phase of life. I knew a woman who told me shortly before her death at 86, "When I retired, I always wanted to volunteer for

Meals on Wheels, but I never did. I wish I had. I don't know what I did daily, but I was busy."

In 2007, Jack Nicholson and Morgan Freeman starred in *The Bucket List*, the story of two terminal cancer patients, old guys, living their last days to the fullest. The film hit a real nerve in our aging Baby Boomer bodies. Since then, "bucket list" has been a common phrase.

An easy way to start a bucket list is to look on the web for bucket-list sites, which often include categories such as fun, possessions, vacations, contributions, spiritual, forgiveness, lifestyle, relationships, adventure, places to visit, personal development, financial, and education.   Under each category that speaks to you, list what comes to mind. Don't hold back. Let your imagination and your dreams soar at this point. If you come up with other categories, add them. Then prioritize your yearnings and add a timeline for when you want to do them. Finally, under each item, list the steps, strategies, and tactics you must take to achievement.

As far as money goes, if you don't think you can afford a dream, consider a different way of doing it. I knew a woman who was a champion bridge player. She went around the world on cruise ships teaching bridge.

What I am concerned more about than money is what I label "analysis paralysis" and "The Censor." By the time I "figure out" lots of stuff, I erroneously conclude that it just can't be done. Then, I find out someone has done it! I suspect that analysis paralysis comes from my censor. This poltergeist, which haunts me, comes out and tells me why—explicitly—I can't do something. I have learned to tell my censor to get lost!

<u>**Time Management**</u>

"What is your plan to do with this one wild and precious life?" asked American poet Mary Oliver.

"Elizabeth, why did you sign up for a workshop on time management?" I sarcastically asked myself as I parked my car. "You—the queen of time management—haven't you had enough of watching the clock after all those years of getting up at a god-awful hour to exercise, walk the dog and battle the interstate to get to your office at the crack of dawn?"

I shuffle to my chair and continue the sardonic query, "You're retired now and can get up when you want to, do what you want to when you want to. You, Elizabeth, are living the American dream!"

Then, the presenter popped in front of the audience with such power, persuasion, and pleasure that I knew my "stinking thinking" was flavored with our American society's pungent beliefs. The myth I had brought into that room was that ladies of a certain age are not valued, powerful, or dynamic. Therefore, there is no reason for them to be concerned anymore with time management because they do not contribute to society!

I have enjoyed not being tied to a timepiece since I retired. Goal-oriented and hard-driven, I worked to get where I am today financially.

The presenter asked us about our goals and to write three of them down. Goals seemed like a unique idea at this age. Then, I realized I had some, and why not try and achieve them? But, if I was going to achieve them, I needed to get started and set aside time to do so, or they would never come to be.

Thinking back to when I was working, I remembered certain habits that helped me save time, such as these:

- Set aside time each day to work on your goal, and don't schedule anything else during this time.

- The night before, decide what you will do and what you will wear the next day so you don't waste time in the morning. Get your breakfast ready to go.

- Viewing time in "chunks" helps: for example, an hour to do housework, two hours to work on a project, and time for yoga or other physical activities.

- Self-care is vital. Be sure you put yourself first, including getting seven-eight hours of sleep, eating nutritious food, exercising, and whatever spiritual practice you do.

- Take yourself out on a little date each week. It helps to rejuvenate the body, mind, and spirit.

The workshop reenergized me, and I realized that however far down the trail of life I am, every minute counts to the very end.

Homework assignments and a list of resources in the appendix will assist you with this critical planning.

The purpose of this chapter's homework is to pamper yourself, practice saying yes to invitations, start a bucket list if you don't have one, record where you spend your time, and see your wishes and dreams for your future life in pictures. Here are five assignments:

1. The little-personal retreat exercise

Plan a whole day, weekend, or week to pamper you. You can schedule a massage, facial, manicure, pedicure, lunch at a unique restaurant, staying at a bed and breakfast inn, etc.

2. The just-say-yes exercise

Become aware of when people ask you to do something and your automatic response. Practice saying yes and see what happens.

3. The bucket-list exercise

Check out several websites about developing a bucket list. Jot down any ideas that interest you. Review several suggested steps on the site that speak to you the most.

4. The tick-tock-clock exercise

For two days, record what you do each hour. Then total the time.

5. The magical collage exercise

This exercise is my favorite. Get a bunch of magazines that you can cut up. Libraries often have piles of them they are getting rid of and will give them to you if you ask. Get a large poster board, a bottle of white glue, and scissors. Sit on the floor, go through the magazines, and cut out any images or words that strike you. Then, arrange them on the poster board and glue them however you want. Step back. Most likely, your wishes, dreams, and future life are staring you in your face. (I have never known this exercise to fail.) Put the board where you will see it every day.

RESOURCES

<u>**Suggested Guidelines for Group Discussions**</u>:

1) Focus on solutions.

2) Avoid cross-talking.

3) Keep comments brief.

4) Refrain from judgment.

<u>Books</u>

Arnaudin, Jess. *Plant-Based Beauty: The Essential Guide to Detoxing Your Beauty Routine.* Piscataway, NJ: Aster, 2019.

Barletta, Marti. *PrimeTime Women.* Chicago, IL: Kaplan Press, 2007.

Beattie, Melody. *More Language of Letting Go: 366 New Daily Meditation.* Center City, MN: Hazelden, 2000.

Breathnach, Sarah Ban. *Simple Abundance: A Daybook of Comfort and Joy.* New York, NY: Grand Central Publishing, 2000.

Cameron, Julia. *The Artist's Way: A Spiritual Path to Higher Creativity.* New York: G. P. Putnam's Sons, 1992.

Cameron, Julia. *It's Never Too Late to Begin Again: Discovering Creativity and Meaning at Midlife and Beyond.* New York: TarcherPerigee, 2016.

Chopra, Deepok MD, *Perfect Health: The Complete Mind Body Guide.* New York, NY: Three Rivers Press, 1991, 2000.

Douglas, Susan J. *In Our Prime: How Older Women Are Reinventing the Road Ahead.* New York, NY: W. W. Norton & Co, 2020.

Gates, Rolf and Kenison, Katrina. *Meditations from the Mat: Daily Reflections on the Path of Yoga.* New York: Anchor Books, 2002.

Gawande, Atul MD, *Being Mortal: Medicine and What Matters in the End.* New York, NY: Metropolitan Books, 2014.

Greenberg, Elinor Miller and Whitney, Fay Wadsworth. *A Time of Our Own in Celebration of Women Over Sixty.* Golden, CO: Fulcrum, 2008.

Kondo, Marie. *The Life-Changing Magic of Tidying Up: The Japanese Art of Decluttering and Organizing.* Berkeley, CA: Ten Speed Press, 2014.

Northrup, Christiane MD, *Women's Bodies, Women's Wisdom: Creating Physical and Emotional Health and Healing.* New York, NY: Bantam, 2020.

Northrup, Christiane MD, *Creating Physical and Emotional Health During the Time of Change.* New York, NY: Bantam, 2012.

Northrup, Christiane MD, *Goddesses Never Age: The Secret Prescription for Radiance, Vitality, and Well-Being.* Carlsbad, CA: Hay House, 2016.

Orman, Suze. *Women and Money: Owning the Power to Control your Destiny.* New York, NY: Spiegel and Grau, 2007.

Pipher, Mary. *Women Rowing North: Navigating Life's Currents and Flourishing As We Age.* New York, NY: Bloomsbury Publishing, 2020.

Sheehy, Gail. *New Passages: Mapping Your Life Across Time.* New York, NY: Ballantine Books, 1996.

Shellenbarger, Sue. *The Breaking Point: How Female Midlife Crisis is Transforming Today's Women.* New York, NY: Henry Holt and Co., 2005.

White-Esmonde, Miranda. *Forever Painless: End Chronic Pain and Reclaim Your Life in Thirty Minutes a Day (Aging Backwards).* 2016.

Winfrey, Oprah. *The Path Made Clear: Discovering Your Life's Direction and Purpose.* New York, NY: Flatiron Books, 2019.

<u>Online Articles</u>

"A New Stretch of the River: Learning to Age with New Openness in Our Hearts and Minds," by Mary Pipher, March/April 2018, psychotherapynetworker.org.

"Getting Enough Protein May Be the Key to Healthy Aging," by Marygrace Taylor, March 14, 2019, prevention.com.

"Americans Are Over Tested, Over Diagnosed and Over Medicated," by Melanie Wiseman, April 2021, beaconseniornews.com.

"Mayo Clinic Q and A: The Health Benefits of Yoga," by Cynthia Weiss, December 28, 2020, mayoclinic.com.

"Breaking Down All the Types of Yoga," by Laura Bennett, January 21, 2021, oola.com.

"6 Popular Yoga Styles Broken Down For Newbies," by Laurel Leicht, aaptiv.com.

"Alcoholism in the Elderly," by Sally K. Rigler, MD, March 15, 2000, American Family Physician, aafp.org.

"Suicide Statistics," 2019, American Foundation for Suicide Prevention, afsp.org.

"The Aging Mouth – and How to Keep It Younger," *Harvard Health Letter,* Harvard Medical School, January, 2010, health.harvard.edu.

"Dehydration - Symptoms and Causes - Mayo Clinic," September 19, 2019, mayoclinic.org.

"Drink Up: Dehydration is an Often Overlooked Health Risk for Seniors – Health Essentials from Cleveland Clinic," November 29, 2018, health.clevelandclinic.org.

"What to do about pelvic organ prolapse - Harvard Health," July 2, 2020, (https:health.harvard.edu.)

"Eleven Hidden Costs of Buying a Home," by Rory Arnold, November 16, 2020, mywallet joy.com.

"The Relocation Decision," by Jane Bryant Quinn – AARP Bulletin, 2016, aarp.org.

" 8 Questions To Help You Decide Whether To Move In Retirement," David Rae, Contributor, October 10, 2018, forbes.com.

"Where to Live After Retirement," by Mary Ann Lawroski, May 8 and June 30, 2014, elderthink.com.

"Mortgages for Seniors: Everything You Need to Know," by Bob Musinski, Contributor, June 11, 2019, *U.S. News and World Report*, loansusnew.com.

"10,000+ Bucket List Ideas For Designing Your Best Life," by Marelisa Fabregia, daringtolivefully.com.

"10 Steps to Help You Plan to Achieve What's on Your Bucket List, " by Jennifer Thompson, June 2, 2020, sixtyandme.com.

Ladies-of-a-Certain-Age Blog Posts

ladiesofacertainage.com

February 13 2013	The Day I Knew I Became Invisible
March 3 2013	Crones – Coming Full Circle
October 2020	The Fifth Circle of Life
August 6 2013	Health, Docs and Pills
April 2019	Health – What If?
February 2016	That Loving Touch
December 2017	Mickey Mouse and I Wish You a Cup of Kindness Cheer
February 2015	Makeup and Herbs –What the ???
March 2014	Taxes and Finances – Really at this age?! – Oh, Please!!!
July 2017	It's 3.a.m. in the Morning. Do you Know Where Your Money Is?
June 2020	A House for the Latter Third of Life
May 2019	U-Hauls Are Not Allowed in Heaven
April 2016	The Ramifications of Spring Cleaning
July 2013	When Are You Moving?
May 2013	Time and TLC – Tender Loving Care
June 2013	Just Say "Yes!"
January 2014	No New Year's Resolutions at this Age – Just a Bucketful of Dreams
October 2014	Friends
August 2017	Add the Final One-Third Cup of Life
May 2018	Got any Change?
November 2018	Don't Give Up Your Power Just Because You Are a Lady-of-a-Certain- Age
August 2018	Time Management – More Important Than 79Ever as We Trot Off into the Sunset

ABOUT THE AUTHOR

Elizabeth was born in Denver on March 29, 1947, and has been igniting the world ever since. Her parents called her Reddy Kilowatt, after the famous utility company mascot, who also had red hair.

She was one of a few women who graduated from the University of Colorado School of Business in 1973 with a graduate degree in marketing. Before retiring, she headed up marketing/public relations departments for two large healthcare nonprofit organizations, a pharmaceutical company, and a hospital.

In addition, Elizabeth had her own company, Ask GENIE Communications! The company focused on educating old house owners about the care of their homes and helping those with historically designated houses obtain Historic Preservation Tax Credits. Passionate about old dwellings, Elizabeth started Denver's Old House Society. The organization offered guided walking tours and an old house fair attended by hundreds each year.

Besides *Paths – A Primer for Ladies-of-a-Certain-Age,* Elizabeth has authored a psychological thriller series, ladies-of-a-certain-age mysteries:` *Murder and Pink Blossoms, Murder and a Victory Garden,* and *Murder and a Blue Spruce.* Her e-newsletter and blog, "Ladies-of-a-Certain-Age," is read by women throughout the United States and several foreign countries. Other books she has authored include two with the late Carole Harshman, *The Fabulous Old Houses of North Seventh Street, Grand Junction, Colorado,* and *A Walking Tour Guidebook to the North Seventh Street Historic Residential District, Grand Junction, Colorado;* and two memoirs, *'57—Memories of a 10-year-old Denver Girl,* and *My Recipe Box.*

Elizabeth has three children and three grandchildren. Currently, she resides on the Western Slope of Colorado with her Airedale Terrier mix, Dolly, and her tuxedo cat, Katie Lane Lynch, named after Elizabeth's great-great-grandmother, an early Colorado pioneer, who is buried in Glenwood Springs, Colorado's Rosebud Cemetery. Elizabeth enjoys gardening, knitting, hiking, and playing pickleball.